# GLUTEN FREE DIET

Breathtaking Recipes for Your Gluten Free Cooking

(Easy and Delicious Gluten Free Recipes for Beginners)

**John Gray**

Published by Sharon Lohan

© **John Gray**

All Rights Reserved

*Gluten Free Diet: Breathtaking Recipes for Your Gluten Free Cooking (Easy and Delicious Gluten Free Recipes for Beginners)*

**ISBN 978-1-990334-14-6**

All rights reserved. No part of this guide may be reproduced in any form without permission in writing from the publisher except in the case of brief quotations embodied in critical articles or reviews.

**Legal & Disclaimer**

The information contained in this book is not designed to replace or take the place of any form of medicine or professional medical advice. The information in this book has been provided for educational and entertainment purposes only.

The information contained in this book has been compiled from sources deemed reliable, and it is accurate to the best of the Author's knowledge; however, the Author cannot guarantee its accuracy and validity and cannot be held liable for any errors or omissions. Changes are periodically made to this book. You must consult your doctor or get professional medical advice before using any of the suggested remedies, techniques, or information in this book.

## Table of contents

Part 1 .................................................................................................. 1

Introduction ...................................................................................... 2

Chapter 1: Definition of Gluten ..................................................... 3

Chapter 2: Is Gluten Required? ..................................................... 6

Chapter 3: Gluten Intolerance ....................................................... 8

Chapter 4: What Does Gluten-Free Eating Look Like? ............ 12

Chapter 5: Breakfast Recipes ....................................................... 16

BREAKFAST .................................................................................... 17

1. Blueberry Pancake Recipe ....................................................... 17

2. Scrambled Eggs with Cilantro and Cheddar ........................ 19

3. Gluten-Free Waffles .................................................................. 21

4. Banana and Strawberry Muffins ............................................ 23

5. Bananas with Coconut Milk .................................................... 25

6. Gluten-Free Butter Milk Doughnut ....................................... 26

Chapter 6: Lunch Recipes ............................................................. 28

7. Potato and Mackerel Salad with Lemon Caraway Dressing
................................................................................................... 28

8. Rice Noodles with Sundried Tomatoes, Parmesan and Basil ....................................................................................... 30

9. Sundried Tomato Bread .................................................. 32

10. Malted Walnut Seed Loaf ............................................. 34

11. Carrot, Pistachio and Feta Salad ................................. 36

12. Roasted Veggies, Quinoa and Feta Cheese Salad ....... 38

Chapter 7: Dinner Recipes ................................................. 40

13. Turkey and Poblano Chili ............................................ 40

14. Chicken with White Beans .......................................... 42

15. Tuna with Black Pepper and Artichokes .................... 44

16. Curried rice and Shrimps ............................................ 46

Chapter 8: Snack Recipes .................................................. 48

17. Spicy Chickpeas ........................................................... 48

18. Halloumi and Bacon Rolls ........................................... 50

19. Sweet and Spicy Popcorn ............................................ 52

20. Salmon and Lemon Mini Fish Cakes .......................... 53

21. Sesame and Chilli Pancakes with Tzatziki ................. 55

22. Skewered Melon and Prosciutto ................................. 57

Chapter 9: Dessert Recipes .................................................. 58

23. Chocolate Pots ............................................................ 58

24. Flourless Chocolate Cake ............................................ 60

25. Maple Baked Apples .................................................. 62

26. Coconut Rice Custard ................................................ 64

27. Raspberry Sorbet and Meringue ............................... 66

Conclusion ........................................................................ 67

Part 2 ................................................................................. 68

Introduction ...................................................................... 69

Gluten Free Diet: A Comprehensive Understanding ....... 71

What Is It? ......................................................................... 71

Why Avoid Gluten? ........................................................... 71

Eat This Not That .............................................................. 73

What To Eat ...................................................................... 73

What To Avoid .................................................................. 74

Breakfast Recipes ............................................................. 77

Gluten-Free Oatmeal ....................................................... 77

Ham & Egg Loaded Potato Skins ..................................... 79

Hash with Poached Eggs ............................................................. 81

Avocado & Bacon Muffins ........................................................... 84

Portobello Breakfast Bakes ......................................................... 86

Classic Breakfast Casserole ........................................................ 88

Brown Fried Rice Breakfast-Style ................................................ 91

Almond Vanilla Scones ............................................................... 93

Lunch Recipes ............................................................................ 95

Chinese Chicken Salad ................................................................ 95

Mediterranean Fish ..................................................................... 98

Tandoori Tofu ............................................................................ 100

Mayo Steak Salad ...................................................................... 102

Sea Vegetable Salad .................................................................. 104

Kale and Fruit Salad-snack ....................................................... 107

Quinoa Burgers ......................................................................... 110

Egg Salad Sandwich .................................................................. 113

Dinner Recipes .......................................................................... 115

Prosciutto-Wrapped Basil Shrimp ............................................. 115

Black-Bean Chili with Winter Squash ........................................ 117

Indian Mushroom Curry ........................................................... 120

Ground Beef Stroganoff ........................................................... 123

Baja Butternut Squash Soup ..................................................... 125

Polenta & Feta Vegetable Medley ............................................... 128

Sweet Potato & Black Bean Chili ................................................ 131

Snack Recipes ........................................................................ 134

The Chewy Gluten Free ............................................................ 134

Fresh Corn Salad .................................................................... 137

Soft-Boiled Egg ....................................................................... 139

Baked Onion Bhajis ................................................................. 141

Barbecue Zucchini Chips ......................................................... 143

Spicy Wedged Sweet Potatoes ................................................... 145

Conclusion ............................................................................. 147

# Part 1

## Introduction

Gluten-free living has been gaining rapid popularity among a wide section of society in recent years owing to several actors among other individuals. This lifestyle is an absolute must for those suffering from gluten intolerance especially those who have been diagnosed with celiac disease. With more than 2 million Americans suffering from varying degrees of celiac diseases, no wonder that the concept of gluten-free living has been spiraling in its acceptance. Additionally, eliminating gluten from the diet has also proven as an effective means of weight loss.

However, before considering adopting gluten-free living, it is essential that we understand the science and applicability of this concept. There are several benefits associated with gluten which may be denied to your body when taking such recourse. Hence complete knowledge of all associated aspects and factors is vital to making an informed decision which can have significant impact on your health and life.

# Chapter 1: Definition of Gluten

**What is Gluten?**

The name gluten is derived from a Latin word which means Glue. It is a protein composite that is usually found in processed food made from wheat. It can even be derived from similar grains like barley and rye. The important property of gluten is that it gives the dough elasticity and allows it to rise and retain its shape. The final product gets the chewy texture because of gluten. Sometimes, it is also used in cosmetics, hair products and dermatological products.

Gluten is composed of *gliadin and glutenin* which is found in several grass like grains, combined with starch. In sources like wheat, about 80% of the protein found in it is made from prolamin and glutelin. True gluten is only found in grass and a few plants from the grass family. Although the proteins stored in maize and similar foods are called glutens, they are not true gluten.

**Extraction of Gluten**

In flour, gluten can be extracted by kneading the gluten into dough and removing the starch. Usually starch granules can be removed with cold water. It is possible to obtain a purer protein by using a saline solution as the harmful impurities are eliminated along with the starch.

In large industries, it is possible to create wheat flour slurry by vigorously kneading the flour with the help of dedicated machines. Then the gluten becomes one large mass that can be collected through centrifugation. It can be transported through several integrated processes that follow.

It is possible to extract close to 65% of the wet gluten with the help of a screw press and the remaining is extracted in a dry chamber.

**Uses of Gluten**

Gluten that is extracted can be put to several uses:

**Bread Production**- Most baked goods make use of gluten as it helps in the process of forming the dough. Yeast is used to raise the dough by releasing carbon dioxide molecules in the form of bubbles. These bubbles are trapped by the gluten molecules making the dough rise. Gluten also helps bind water through hydration to keep the shape of the dough.

**Imitation Meats:** Gluten derived from wheat is most often used to produce imitation meat that resembles beef, chicken, duck and fish. This meat, when cooked, becomes firm to bite as the gluten absorbs the moisture surrounding the meat.

**Other Foods:** Gluten can also be used in several other food products like beer and soy sauce. It is used as a stabilizing product in certain foods like ketchup and ice cream.

**Animal Feed:** In some pet foods, their quality is enhanced with the use of gluten.

# Chapter 2: Is Gluten Required?

Before delving into the intricacies of gluten-free living it is essential to understand its effects on the human body both in the positive as well as negative aspects. Those who are gluten intolerant can have several health issues on consuming this product. However, for those whose body is accepting of gluten, consuming foods that contain gluten may actually have some health benefits. The truth is that gluten is mostly found in whole grains. While there are no real nutritional benefits from gluten itself, consuming these foods can provide you with several vitamins and minerals. Whole grains and similar products can considerably lower the risk of heart attacks and also type-2 diabetes. Most of our carbohydrates also come from whole grain products. The advantages of including gluten in our diet are:

**High Protein Source**

You can get 50% of the recommended protein intake with just one 4 ounce serving of gluten. Although the protein content is so high, the amount of fat contained in it is negligible. For example, a ¼ cup of wheat provides 23 grams of protein and just 0.5 grams of fat.

**High Source of Iron**

Gluten consists of a high percentage of iron. In just ¼ cup of wheat, you can acquire 9% iron.

**Other Nutrients**

Other nutrients like calcium may be derived from gluten. The primary advantage is that gluten does not add any cholesterol to the body while adding these nutrients.

It is recommended that people who do not eat meat should consume gluten. It can be a valuable source of proteins. Even those who are allergic to dairy can consume gluten to get their share of proteins. Additionally if you are on a strict low fat and low-carb diet, gluten can be a great dietary inclusion for you. When you consume the right amount of gluten, you feel energetic, yet extremely light.

However all this doesn't make Gluten an absolute necessity in your diet and it does have a whole lot of negative influence on your body systems in case you have Gluten intolerance.

# Chapter 3: Gluten Intolerance

Gluten Intolerance or gluten sensitivity includes a spectrum of eating disorders related to gluten. The most common disease is celiac disease which is a very strong immune reaction to glucose resistance. This condition usually begins at the stage of infancy leading to extreme diarrhea, weight loss and continuous fatigue. In most people, unfortunately, this condition is asymptomatic. This means that there are no symptoms of the disease at all, making it very hard to diagnose.

Celiac Disease is usually a reaction to a protein named gliadin that is a constituent of gluten. This protein is mostly found in barley, wheat and rye. Some doctors also recommend that people who have celiac disease should stay clear of oats as well.

The consequences of celiac disease include- inflammation and rupture of the inner small intestine lining. This is actually an allergic reaction that occurs when gluten is included in the diet. The reason for this chronic disorder is reduced absorption of necessary minerals and nutrients.

As per most medical examiners, there is no definite cure for this condition. It can, however, be kept under control with effective treatment and a complete gluten- free diet.

**Symptoms of Celiac Disease**

The most common symptoms include:

- Persistent stomach ache
- Development of external symptoms like rashes
- Extreme Fatigue
- Anemia
- Abdominal Discomfort like gas and bloating

Celiac Disease is a permanent disorder. As a result, the effects of the disease can continuously change with time. Sometimes there are associated symptoms like irregular bowel movements. The symptom itself can vary greatly from mild to severe. It is also possible that you never experience any symptom at all.

There are several other diseases that have similar symptoms. Therefore, it is important to have your condition diagnosed first to make sure that you are gluten resistant. Celiac disease can be diagnosed with the help of blood tests and also a small intestine biopsy.

## Treatment for Celiac Disease

In most cases, the only solution to gluten intolerance is avoiding gluten completely. All products that can contain even traces of Gluten should be eliminated from the diet entirely. Observing a gluten-free diet strictly gives your intestines a chance to heal completely. With a change in the way you eat, it is possible to end all the noticeable symptoms entirely.

You must be completely aware of the foods that are safe for you and the foods that might be hazardous. You can even consume vitamin and mineral supplements to reduce further health issues that may be caused by a gluten-free diet.

## Other Gluten Related Health Disorders

There are several other health disorders besides Celiac disease that can arise due to gluten resistance. They include:

- **Dermititis Herpetiformis:** This disorder is accompanied by itchy rashes and extremely painful blisters and bumps on the skin. It usually occurs on the elbows, knees, scalp and back.

- **Gluten Ataxia:** Those who are genetically susceptible to gluten sensitivity may experience this disorder. The common symptoms include inability of the brain to regulate limb strength and movement.

- **Non Celiac Gluten Sensitivity:** This disorder has also been termed as gluten hypersensitivity. Abdominal Discomfort, extreme fatigue, lethargy, muscle cramps and headaches are the common symptoms of this disorder.

**What causes Gluten Sensitivity?**

In most people, gluten can cause gluten toxicity. The constituents of gluten increase the permeability of the intestinal cells resulting in abdominal discomfort. There are also some receptors in these constituents that destroy the tight junctions around the cells. These junctions are responsible for the prevention of leakage around the cells that line the small intestine. As a result, food proteins leak into the body causing various symptoms.

# Chapter 4: What Does Gluten-Free Eating Look Like?

A gluten-free diet refers to a meal plan that excludes the protein - gluten. This complex protein is mostly found in wheat, rye and triticale. Usually a gluten-free diet is only recommended as an effective treatment for celiac disease. There are several other gluten intolerance related issues that can be cured with the help of a simple gluten-free diet.

There has been a significant increase in the demand for gluten-free food in the last couple of years with gluten-free eating emerging as a 'fad' among the fitness conscious people.

**Gluten-Free Foods**

There are several grains and other starch sources that work well in a gluten-free diet. These foods include potatoes, tapioca, rice and even corn. You can even consume grains like montina, lupin, quinoa, sorghum and chia seeds in your gluten-free diet. Beans like soya bean and nut flours can be included in the diet to provide dietary fiber.

If you are picking foods from stands, then you must be very careful in checking the gluten-free labels on them. There are several foods like ketchup where we least expect the inclusion of gluten. However, it may be included in the form of a stabilizing agent. So, make sure you read the label before you pick up any type of processed food.

You can include fresh fruits and vegetables in your diet. You can also add fat sources like butter and margarine without any worry.

**Health Hazards of Gluten-Free Diet**

Although gluten-free diet is recommended only for those with evident gluten related issues, there are several regular individuals who practice this diet. While the health benefits of removing gluten from your diet are plenty, you may also have adverse health effects if you do not follow the diet correctly.

Gluten containing foods like whole grains are extremely rich in minerals and vitamins that are essential for our body. If you decide to follow a gluten-free diet, you must make it a point to consume necessary supplements to make up for the lack of these nutrients. This reduces the risk of deficiency related disorders.

However, there is actually no real need to take the risk of eliminating gluten if you have no issues. If you still insist, make sure you do it right to enjoy the benefits.

**Health Benefits of a Gluten-Free Diet**

For those who are suffering from gluten sensitivity, this is the only treatment available. The symptoms and discomfort related to gluten can only be eliminated by removing it entirely from the diet. Of course, the popularity of gluten-free foods at grocery stores is increasing tremendously. This is because a gluten-free diet may have additional health benefits to even regular people.

When you consume gluten-free food, the amount of cholesterol in your body is reduced significantly. Additionally, gluten is a complex protein which means that it is difficult to digest. It takes time to be broken down for consumptions. As a result, substituting gluten with simpler proteins can improve digestion and hence promote gastrointestinal health.

**Beware of Cross Contamination**

Whenever you adopt a gluten-free diet, make sure you check for cross contamination. This occurs when gluten-free food comes in contact with foods containing gluten. This contamination may occur during the manufacturing process. Sometimes, the same equipment may be used to produce gluten-free food and also process food containing gluten. The only way to make sure that you do not suffer due to cross contamination is to check for a label that says 'May contain gluten'.

When you are unsure of the food you are buying, don't buy it at all. If need be, you could check with the manufacturer before making the purchase. It is also possible to cross contaminate food while cooking at home. So be very careful to use separate dishes for gluten-free ingredients and ingredients containing gluten.

# Chapter 5: Breakfast Recipes

When you need to go completely gluten-free, it might seem like your food options are reduced significantly. The truth is that there are several gluten-free substitutes that you can add to your cooking to make delicious gluten-free meals. Here are some fun recipes that you can include in your scrumptious gluten-free meal plan.

# BREAKFAST

## 1. Blueberry Pancake Recipe

Ingredients:

Gluten-Free Flour- 1¼ cups (it is advised to add some xanthan gum)

Organic Cane Sugar- 2 tablespoons

Gluten-Free Baking Powder- 1 teaspoon

Baking Soda- 1 teaspoon

Egg- 1 large

Olive Oil- 2 Tablespoons

Buttermilk- 1 1/4$^{th}$ Cup

Fresh Blueberries- 1 cup

Vegetable Oil- to fry the pancakes

Procedure:

Mix all the dry ingredients in a bowl and whisk them together

Beat the eggs separately till they are thick. Add some oil and buttermilk and blend them

Now add all the dry ingredients and mix them together to make a batter. Stir in the blueberries

On a heavy skillet add a tsp of oil and pour in about 3/4$^{th}$ Cup and smooth the pancake. When the bottom is golden brown, just flip the pancake and let it fry completely.

Serve the pancakes with a little maple syrup.

## 2. Scrambled Eggs with Cilantro and Cheddar

Ingredients

Eggs- 4 large

Olive oil- 1 tablespoon

Chopped Onion- ¼ the Cup

Diced Tomato- 1 medium sized

Cilantro- 2-4 tablespoons

Salt

Ground Black Pepper

Low Fat Shredded Cheddar- $1/4^{th}$ Cup

Procedure

Whisk the eggs with 2 Tablespoons until they blend well.

Warm the olive oil on a large skillet

Cook the onions in the oil until they are golden brown.

Now, cook the tomatoes and the cilantro. Add a dash of black pepper. Make sure all the juice from the tomato is completely dry.

Reduce the flame and pour the eggs over the cooked vegetables. Cook the eggs without stirring them for a while. Then, stir the edges of the eggs towards the centre of the skillet.

Let the eggs cook for a while. When they are still moist but almost cooked, you can add the cheddar cheese.

Once the eggs are completely cooked, divide and serve them.

## 3. Gluten-Free Waffles

### Ingredients

Brown Rice or Rice Flour- 1 cup

Potato Starch- ½ Cup

Baking Powder- 2 teaspoons

Tapioca Flour- ¼ Cup

Salt

Oil- ¼ Cup

Eggs- 2

Buttermilk- 1 ½ Cup

Sugar- 1 Teaspoon

### Procedure

Mix all the ingredients together and whisk them well.

If the mixture is not of pouring consistency, just add some milk.

Pour the batter into a waffle iron and serve warm.

You can serve it with maple syrup or chocolate syrup.

## 4. Banana and Strawberry Muffins

Ingredients

Rice Flour- 1 ¼ cup

Potato Starch- 1/4th Cup

Tapioca Flour- ¼ Cup

Xanthan Gum- ½ teaspoon

Powdered Cinnamon- ¼ spoon

Baking Powder- 1 ½ Teaspoons

Salt to taste

Butter or Margarine- ½ Cup

Sugar- 1/3 Cup

Eggs- 2

Pure Vanilla Extract- ½ teaspoon

Milk- 1/3 Cup

Peeled Bananas- 2

Stemmed and Chopped Strawberries- 1 ½ Cup

## Procedure

Stir the rice flour, potato starch, tapioca flour, xanthan gum, baking soda, baking powder, cinnamon and salt in a bowl. Blend them well.

Cream the butter and Sugar till they are smooth. Then beat the eggs and pour in with vanilla and milk . The mixture might get lumpy.

Fold in the strawberries and mashed bananas into the batter.

Grease Muffin Cups with butter or oil and pour the batter into them.

Bake the batter in an oven preheated to 350°F. Allow the batter to bake for about 30 minutes. Put a skewer in and pull it out.

If it comes out clean, it means that your muffins are ready to serve.

## 5. Bananas with Coconut Milk

Ingredients

Sliced Bananas- 2

Coconut Milk- ¼ Cup

Maple Syrup or honey- 4 tablespoons

Powdered Cinnamon

Procedure

Separate all the slices of bananas in a small bowl

Pour the Coconut milk over the bananas

Drizzle the mixture with honey or maple syrup

Chill and Serve

## 6. Gluten-Free Butter Milk Doughnut

Ingredients

Eggs- 2

Buttermilk- 2 cups

Butter- ¼ Cup

Gluten-Free Rice Flour- 5 Cups

Sugar- 1 Cup

Nutmeg- 1 Teaspoon

Baking Soda- 2 Teaspoons

Baking Powder- 1 Teaspoon

Salt

Xanthan Gum- 2 teaspoons

Sugar- ½ Cup

Procedure

In a large bowl, whisk beaten eggs, buttermilk and butter together.

In a separate bowl mix all the dry ingredients

Slowly fold them into the egg mixture. Knead the dough with your hands and add some flour if you need.

Roll the dough out and cut it with a doughnut cutter.

Take the canola oil in a pan and allow it to heat. Drop the doughnuts into the oil. Cook them till they are completely golden brown. Drain the oil and allow the doughnuts to cool a little.

While they are still warm, roll these doughnuts in sugar and serve.

# Chapter 6: Lunch Recipes

## 7. Potato and Mackerel Salad with Lemon Caraway Dressing

Ingredients

Potatoes- 175g

Smoked Mackerel Fillets with Skin Removed- 200g

Cooked Beetroot, Sliced- 140g

Finely Chopped Dill- 1 bunch

Olive Oil- 2 Tablespoons

Lemon Juice- 1 lemon

Lemon Zest- 1 lemon

Caraway Seeds- 1/4th Teaspoons

Procedure

In a small saucepan, boil the potatoes until they are fork tender

Flake the mackerel and add the potatoes, spring onions, dill and beetroot

For the dressing, mix the olive oil, lemon juice, caraway seeds and some salad seasoning. Pour it over the vegetables and toss them and serve. Scatter the lemon zest to garnish

## 8. Rice Noodles with Sundried Tomatoes, Parmesan and Basil

Ingredients

Rice Noodles- 250g

Sundried tomatoes- 85g

Sundried Tomato Oil- 2 tablespoons

Garlic Cloves- 3

Grated Parmesan- 25g

Basil Leaves- 1 handful

Procedure

Boil the rice noodles and strain them.

Heat oil in a pan.

Fry the sundried tomatoes and garlic for about 3 minutes.

Toss the noodles in the tomatoes and garlic. Add some seasoning and toss in most of the cheese.

Once it is ready, just sprinkle the remaining cheese and basil on the noodles and serve.

## 9. Sundried Tomato Bread

Ingredients

Gluten-free Flour- 200g

Salt

Gluten-Free Baking Powder- 2 tsp

Tomato Puree- 1 tsp

Butter Milk- 284 ml

Eggs- 3

Sundried Tomatoes- 65g

Parmesan, Grated- 25g

Procedure

Preheat the oven to 160°C.

In a large bowl, mix the salt, baking powder and flour

Whisk the buttermilk, eggs, tomato Puree and oil separately.

Fold the dry ingredients in to the wet mixture along with tomatoes and parmesan.

Grease a 900g loaf tin and pour the mixture in.

Sprinkle the remaining Parmesan on the mixture and bake for 60 minutes.

Poke in a skewer after 60 minutes.

If it comes out clean, it is ready to serve.

## 10. Malted Walnut Seed Loaf

<u>Ingredients</u>

Corn flour- 100g

Gluten-Free Brown Bread Flour- 300g

Soya Flour- 2 tablespoons

Potato Starch- 85g

Xanthan Gum- 2 Teaspoons

Easy Bake Dried Yeast- 7g

Caster Sugar- 1 tablespoon

Warm Milk- 450 ml

Sunflower Oil- 2 tablespoons

White Wine Vinegar- 1 tablespoon

Mixed Seeds- 100g

Chopped Walnuts- 50g

<u>Procedure</u>

Mix all the flours, the xanthan gum, yeast, sugar and salt in a large bowl.

In a separate bowl, mix the milk, oil and vinegar.

Fold the dry ingredients into this mixture until they have the consistency of a soft dough.

Cover the dough loosely with cling wrap and allow it to rise for an hour.

When the dough has risen, add the seeds and walnuts into it and knead.

Grease your palm with oil and make a large round shape. Roll this round dough in the remaining seeds and nuts. Cover and leave aside for another hour.

Heat the oven to 200°C. Bake the bread for about 15 minutes.

Reduce the heat to about 190°C and bake the bread for about 30 minutes.

Once it's done, allow it to cool and then cut into slices and serve.

## 11. Carrot, Pistachio and Feta Salad

Ingredients

Olive Oil- 2 tablespoons

Carrots- 500g,

Canned Chickpeas- 400 g

Ground Cumin- 2 Teaspoons

Lemon Juice- ½ lemon

Clear Honey- 1 tablespoon

Shelled Pistachios- 100g

Mint- Small Bunch

Spinach- 2 large handfuls

Crumbled Feta Cheese- 200g

Procedure

Preheat the oven to 200°C. Add some oil, the carrots, chickpeas and cumin into a baking tray. Season and toss and roast for 30 minutes till carrots feel tender.

Mix the lemon juice, honey and oil and pour onto the roasted carrots and chickpeas. You can keep this mixture in the fridge and bring it out an hour before serving.

Toss the Spinach, Mint and Pistachios into this mixture. Check the seasoning, drizzle some oil, sprinkle the feta cheese and serve.

## 12. Roasted Veggies, Quinoa and Feta Cheese Salad

Ingredients

Quinoa- 200 g

Olive Oil- 3 Tablespoons

Red Onion, sliced into thick circles - 1

Chunky pieces of red or yellow peppers- 2 whole

Courgettes, halved lengthways- 200g

Garlic Cloves- 3

Lemon Juice and Zest- 1 lemon

Sugar- one pinch

Roughly Chopped Parsley

Feta Cheese- 200g

Procedure

Cook and drain the quinoa well.

Heat the oven to 200°C. Toss in the onion and peppers with 1 tbsp of oil and seasoning on a roasting tray. Roast this mixture for 15 minutes.

Throw in the courgettes, garlic and remaining veggies and roast for 15 more minutes.

Squeeze the roasted garlic cloves out of their skin. Mash them with some seasoning and stir in the remaining oil, zest and lemon juice.

Drizzle this dressing over the quinoa and mix with the roasted vegetables and parsley.

When you want to serve this dish, just sprinkle the crumbled Feta cheese over it.

# Chapter 7: Dinner Recipes

## 13. Turkey and Poblano Chili

Ingredients

Olive Oil-    1 tablespoon

Chopped Onion- 1 whole

Poblano Pepper, chopped- 1 whole

Ground Cumin – 2 Teaspoons

Diced Tomatoes- 1 Can

Kidney Beans- 2 Cans

Salt

Roasted and Shredded turkey ( you can replace it with chicken)- 2 cups

Procedure

In a large sauce pan, heat the oil on medium flame. Add the onions and Poblano Peppers. Cook until they begin to soften and then add the cumin seeds.

Now add the tomatoes, with the juice. When it begins to boil slightly, add beans and 2 cups of water, salt and pepper. Bring the whole mixture to boil.

Allow the mixture to simmer till it is slightly thickened.

Add the turkey and cook for about 3 minutes.

Serve with tortilla chips.

## 14. Chicken with White Beans

Ingredients

Canned Rinsed Cannellini Beans- 2 cans

Grape Tomatoes- 1 pint

Fresh Thyme- 4 sprigs

Smashed Garlic Cloves- 2

Crushed Garlic- 2 cloves

Fresh Oregano- 4 sprigs

Crushed Red Pepper- ¼ teaspoon

Olive Oil0 2 tablespoons

Salt and Black Pepper

Chicken Thighs- 3 pounds

Procedure

Heat the oven to about 425°F

In a Large baking dish, mix the beans, tomatoes, thyme, oregano sprigs, garlic, red pepper, oil, salt and black pepper.

Pat the chicken dry and place it above the bean mixture. Glaze the chicken with some oil and season with salt and pepper.

Roast this mixture till the chicken is completely cooked and golden. It should take about 35 minutes.

Garnish with oregano leaves and serve.

## 15. Tuna with Black Pepper and Artichokes

Ingredients

Rice- 1 cup

Olive Oil- 2 tablespoons

Red Onion- Thinly Sliced

Drained and Halved Artichoke Hearts- 3 jars

Lemon slices- 8

Sliced Garlic Cloves- 2

Thyme- 4 sprigs

Fresh Tuna, cut into cubes- 1 ½ pounds

Kosher Salt- 1 ½ teaspoons

Black Pepper- 1 Teaspoon

Procedure

Cook the rice completely

On a large skillet, heat some oil. Fry the onions till they become soft

To the onions, add artichokes, lemon, garlic and thyme. Cook them well and transfer to a plate.

Season the tuna with salt and pepper and cook the tuna in some oil in the same skilled. When it is brown on all sides, you can toss in the artichoke mixture.

Serve with cooked rice.

## 16. Curried rice and Shrimps

Ingredients

Olive Oil- 1 tablespoon

Chopped Onion- 1 large

Carrots, chopped- 2

Garlic Cloves- 2

Curry Powder- 2 teaspoons

Long Grain white Rice- 1 cup

Salt and Pepper

Peeled and Deveined large shrimp- 1 ½ pounds

Fresh Basil- 1 ½ cups

Procedure

In a large skillet heat some oil. Cook the onions and carrots in this oil. Stir them until they are soft.

Add garlic and Curry Powder and continue to cook. Stir the mixture till it becomes fragrant.

Add rice and 1 ½ cups of water. Add salt and pepper and bring to boil. Allow the contents to cook, covered for about 15 minutes.

Season the shrimps with salt and pepper and place in the cooked rice. Cover and continue to cook.

When the shrimp is opaque, it is time to fold in the basil and serve your dish.

# Chapter 8: Snack Recipes

**SNACKS**

## 17. Spicy Chickpeas

Ingredients

Drained and Dried Chickpeas- 400g

Vegetable Oil- 1 Teaspoon

Chili Powder- 1 tablespoon

Procedure

In a large bowl, mix the vegetable oil, chili powder and chickpeas.

Make sure the chickpeas are coated with the chili

Transfer the coated chickpeas into a baking sheet and cook them for about 25 minutes.

Allow the chickpeas to cool. You will see that they have become quite crisp.

Just sprinkle some sea salt and enjoy this healthy snack with the family.

## 18. Halloumi and Bacon Rolls

Ingredients

Halloumi Cheese- 250g

Pancetta or Smoked Bacon- 10

Chopped Chives- 1 tablespoon

Procedure

Heat the oven to about 180°C.

Cut the Halloumi cheese into 20 sticks.

Stretch out the bacon or the pancetta using the back of the knife and cut in half.

To season, sprinkle some black pepper and chopped chives onto the pancetta.

Roll the pancetta around the halloumi blocks.

Place them on a baking sheet.

Bake for about 12 minutes.

When the pancetta is brown and crisp, your dish is ready to serve.

## 19. Sweet and Spicy Popcorn

Ingredients

Salted Microwave Popcorn- 100g

Chilli Powder- ¼ tbsp

Cinnamon- ½ teaspoon

Agave Syrup- 1 Tablespoon

Procedure

Cook the microwave popcorn as per the instructions on the packet

Tip the popcorn into a large bowl.

Sprinkle the chili powder and cinnamon over the popcorn and stir well.

Pour the agave sauce over the chilli popcorn and stir.

Serve warm.

## 20. Salmon and Lemon Mini Fish Cakes

Ingredients

Baking potatoes- 2 large

Olive Oil- 2 tablespoons

Lemon zest and Juice- ½ lemon

Egg yolk- 1

Smoked Salmon Trimmings- 140g

Chopped Parsley- 1 tablespoon

Gluten-Free Flour mixed with I tsp coarsely ground pepper- 2 tablespoons

Oil to Fry


Directions

Microwave the potatoes till they are tender.

Allow them to cool for about 5 minutes

Scoop the flesh and mash in a bowl.

Season the mashed potatoes with olive oil, lemon zest and lemon juice.

Mix in the egg, salmon and parsley.

Shape the potato into tiny balls and chill for 15 minutes.

Dust them with flour and fry in a little oil with low heat. Cook till it is golden.

Drain the oil, sprinkle some parsley and serve.

## 21. Sesame and Chilli Pancakes with Tzatziki

Ingredients

For Pancakes:

Gluten-Free Flour- 100 g

Egg- 1 whole

Soya Yoghurt- 1 whole

Green and red chili chopped finely- 1 each

Diced Spring Onions- 1 bunch

Chopped Coriander- 2 tablespoons

Sesame Seeds- 1 tablespoon

For Tzatziki

Greek Yoghurt- 150g

Cucumber, deseeded and grated- 1

Chopped Mint- 1 Tablespoons

Procedure

Make a smooth batter with the eggs, soya yoghurt and 2 tbsp water.

Stir the chilies, spring onions, coriander and sesame seeds.

Allow the mixture to chill.

To make the tzatziki, mix the Greek yoghurt, cucumber and mint together. Add some salt and pepper and allow it t chill.

In a small frying pan, heat a splash of oil.

Add one teaspoonful of pancake mix and smoothen it out. Cook till it is lightly brown. Pile the pancakes onto a plate.

Serve with a dollop of tzatziki and some sliced Spring onions.

## 22. Skewered Melon and Prosciutto

Ingredients

Cantaloupe Melon, cut into bite sized pieces- 1

Prosciutto- 12- 14 Slices

Cocktail Sticks- 40

Procedure

Deseed the cantaloupe and cut it into quarters

Cut it into bite sized pieces.

Cut the prosciutto into 3 long strips each and wrap around the melon pieces.

Secure with the cocktail stick and serve.

# Chapter 9: Dessert Recipes

## 23. Chocolate Pots

Ingredients

Granulated Sugar- 2/3 Cups

Cornstarch- 2 Tablespoons

Kosher Salt

Whole Milk- 3 Cups

Egg Yolks= 4 large

Pure Vanilla Extract- ½ Teaspoon

Bittersweet Chocolate- 6 ounces

Unsweetened Cocoa Powder- ½ teaspoon

Procedure

In a saucepan, mix the sugar and cornstarch. Add some salt. Continue to stir and slowly add 1/3 of the milk into this mixture.

When this forms a smooth paste, beat the eggs and stir them in with the remaining milk.

Use a wooden spoon to stir this mixture. When it is thickened, remove it from the heat.

Add the vanilla and chocolate and continue to stir toll the chocolate melts completely. The mixture should be completely smooth by the end of it.

Pour this mixture into glasses or ramekins.

Cover it and refrigerate for at least two hours. You can leave this in the fridge for a maximum of two days.

Serve with a sprinkling of cocoa powder.

## 24. Flourless Chocolate Cake

### Ingredients

Unsalted Butter, cut into pieces- 1 Cup

Unsweetened Cocoa powder- ¼ Cup

Heavy Cream- 1 ¼ Cup

Chopped Bitter sweet Chocolate- 8 ounces

Large Eggs- 5

Granulated Sugar- 1 Cup

Sour Cream- ½ Cup

Confectioners' Sugar- ¼ Cup

### Procedure

Heat the pan to 350°F.

Butter a springform pan and dust with cocoa powder

In a saucepan, heat the butter with ¼ of the heavy cream till the butter melts completely.

Add the chocolate to this mixture and stir till it is smooth. Remove from heat

In a large bowl, whisk the eggs along with the granulated sugar and cocoa powder. Fold the chocolate mixture in.

Transfer this batter into the pan that you prepared in the beginning. Allow it to bake till it becomes puffed and completely set. This should take about 40 minutes.

Allow the cake to cool. Get the edges off with a knife and unmould it.

In an electric mixer, beat the heavy cream and sour cream with confectioners' sugar till soft peaks are formed.

Sprinkle the remaining confectioners' sugar on the cake and serve with the whipped cream.

## 25. Maple Baked Apples

### Ingredients

Large Apples-4

Maple Syrup- ¾ cup

Walnut Pieces- ½ Cup

Golden Raisins- ¼ Cup

Unsalted Butter- 2 Tablespoons

Ice cream- Optional

### Procedure

Heat the oven to 400°F

Remove the core of the apple and trim about ½ inch slices from the bottom of the apple so it can sit flat.

Place the apples in an 8-9 inch baking dish.

Drizzle them with some syrup.

Fill the cavities in the apples with raisins and walnuts. Keep the remaining to garnish.

Dot the apples with butter and bake for 40-50 minutes till they are completely tender.

Pour the liquid from the baking dish into a skillet. In a medium saucepan, bring this liquid to boil. Allow it to thicken slightly.

Pour the sauce over the warm apples and serve with some ice cream.

## 26. Coconut Rice Custard

Ingredients

Unsweetened Coconut Milk- 1 Can

Water- ¼ Cup

Sugar- ½ Cup + 2/3 Cup

Long Grain White Rice- 1 Cup

Half and Half- 3 Cups

Eggs- 5

Vanilla Extract- 1 Teaspoon

Procedure

Heat the oven to 325°F.

In a saucepan, bring the coconut milk, water and ¼ Cup sugar to boil.

Stir the rice in. In a low flame, cover and allow it to simmer. When the rice is tender and all the liquid is absorbed, turn off the heat. This will take about 20 minutes.

In another saucepan, warm the half and half. Make sure it does not boil.

In a bowl, whisk the eggs, vanilla and the rest of the sugar.

Continue to whisk your mixture and pour the warm half and half into it. Skim off any foam that may form on the surface. You can discard this foam as it is of no use to the preparation.

Now, stir the rice in.

Transfer all the contents into an 8 inch baking dish.

Place this dish in a larger pan.

Now add hot water carefully into the larger pan. The water must come up half way up the sides of the smaller dish.

Bake until the custard is fully set. It will take about an hour.

You can serve it cold or warm as per your preference.

## 27. Raspberry Sorbet and Meringue

Ingredients

Heavy Cream- 1 Cup

Confectioners' Sugar- 2 Tablespoons

Meringue Cookies- 16

Raspberry Sorbet- 2 Pints

Procedure

Whip the cream and sugar in a medium bowl. You must continue to whisk till medium peaks are formed. Set this aside.

Break the cookies and tip into another medium sized bowl.

In individual dishes, scoop the raspberry sorbet.

Spoon the whipped cream over the sorbet and sprinkle the crumbled cookies over them.

Serve chilled.

# Conclusion

The biggest possible challenge with a gluten-free diet is sticking to it. But with so many recipes at hand, it is definitely a lot easier now. As you indulge in new recipes and cooking techniques, you will wonder why you never considered going gluten-free before. You will notice a considerable change in your energy levels which will help you get through your day better. You will observe that your sleep pattern also gets better as you make your diet gluten-free and light.

You can pick several ingredients that are completely gluten- free to experiment on your own. If you still find it hard to stick to your diet, make a simple chart that tells you what to cook on each day of the week. Avoid eating out whenever possible. You can never be entirely sure that the restaurants serve 100% gluten-free food, even when they claim to.

# Part 2

## Introduction

This book has actionable information that will help you to follow a gluten free diet effortlessly by preparing mouth watering gluten free recipes.

Wheat is undoubtedly one of the most commonly used ingredients in many American kitchens and perhaps around the world. From being used as a thickening agent to being used to make cakes, bread, cookies and a host of other delicious foods, wheat seems to be just one of those products that we almost cannot live without.

But do you know that the wheat that you are so passionate about using could perhaps be the one thing that has been causing you many of the problems you might be having? From skin rashes to gas and constipation to diarrhea and a host of other problems, wheat can cause all that. Have you noticed that you have an upset stomach or experience different digestive problems after eating foods containing wheat? From cakes to bread and beer to cookies, is it that you just cannot 'stomach' foods made of wheat, barley and rye?

The question that might be running through your mind right now could be; so what's with wheat that makes it so bad? One word; GLUTEN! The gluten found in **wheat, rye and barley** is the root of all evil that follows after you've taken products containing such ingredients. The problem could be so bad that you could suffer from an autoimmune disease referred from celiac disease, a genetic condition where the lining of your gut is damaged by the effects of gluten on your digestive system. Lucky for you, this book has information that will help you to understand gluten better, as well as how to avoid it. And to top it off, you will discover some delicious recipes guaranteed to help you to stay off gluten effortlessly.

# Gluten Free Diet: A Comprehensive Understanding

### What Is It?

A gluten free diet is simply a diet that does not contain gluten.

Gluten is a type of protein found in grains such as barley, wheat, rye and triticale (a cross between rye and wheat). It is what gives these products their gluey/sticky nature hence making them key ingredients for baking where elasticity of dough is required.

The thing is, gluten contains up to 80% of all proteins found in wheat and basically nourishes the embryo of wheat seeds during germination. But despite wheat being delicious, gluten has a low nutritional value. Moreover, the grains that contain gluten aren't essential in your diet.

So what is so wrong that you want to avoid it anyway?

### Why Avoid Gluten?

In addition to being less nutritious, the gluten in wheat, barley or rye isn't properly digested into amino acids like other proteins. This is because the protein breaks down in various peptides or short strings of amino acids, which can't be further broken down.

And if you suffer from celiac disease, each peptide reacts in a manner that it increases the toxicity of other peptides. Celiac disease is a serious autoimmune response caused by gluten consumption, and is characterized by bloody or fatty stools, nausea, gas, diarrhea, stomach pain as well as appetite changes. Sensitivity to gluten can lead to symptoms that correspond to celiac disease such as breathing problems, diarrhea, vomiting, facial swelling, hives and itchy rashes. Most of these symptoms occur because gluten causes *inflammation* in your small intestines especially if you are gluten intolerant or suffer from celiac disease. The immune system responds to invaders like viruses, germs, bacteria and allergens such as gluten through inflammation. Unfortunately, the inflammatory response may cause toxins and microbes to buildup in the blood stream leading to chronic inflammation. If that happens, your entire body system gets overwhelmed, and it sends incorrect signals about what invaders to be destroyed. At the end, your immune system ends up destroying its own cells in what is referred to as *autoimmune disease*.

If diagnosed with celiac disease, adapting a gluten-free diet can help reduce the autoimmune reactions and prevent hazardous complications.

Here's how to go about it:

# Eat This Not That

### What To Eat

While you might find the gluten free diet frustrating to adopt initially, you will find comfort in knowing that there are many foods that are already gluten free. All you need to do is substitute the ones with the gluten and enjoy!

Many healthy and delicious foods such as fresh eggs, fresh meats, beans and most dairy products are naturally gluten free. However, be sure that these are not mixed or processed with gluten containing additives, grains or preservative when you purchase them.

Here's a comprehensive list of what you can eat:

- Fresh eggs

- Fruits and vegetables

- Fresh meats, fish and poultry; but not marinated, batter-coated or breaded

- Unprocessed beans, seeds and nuts

- Most dairy products such as plain ice cream, plain yogurt, real cheese, margarine, butter and milk

- Starches and grains such as buckwheat, arrow root, corn and cornmeal, amaranth, rice, quinoa, millet, sorghum and soy

- Distilled vinegar but not malt vinegar

- Distilled alcoholic drinks where gluten is removed during processing

- Natural spices like garlic, ginger, cinnamon etc.

- Buckwheat

- Flours and baked goods made from gluten-free products such as rice, almonds etc

## What To Avoid

Eating a gluten-free diet can help you control the signs and symptoms of celiac disease, as well as prevent hazardous complications caused by gluten intolerance. Avoid the following foods:

- Wheat varieties such as spelt, kamut
- Breads, cakes, candies, cereal, cookies and French fries unless labeled as gluten-free
- Rye, mostly found in bread products
- Barley and beers such as malt vinegar, malt flavoring and malt.
- Semolina
- Graham flour
- Farina
- Durum flour
- Licorice or candies made with barley or wheat
- Modified wheat starch, though can be considered gluten-free f processed to remove gluten
- Oats grown alongside wheat or barley; unless the oat product is labeled gluten-free.
- Processed cheese such as spray cheese

- Marinade or sauce that has added gluten such as teriyaki sauce.

If you're gluten intolerant or if at risk of celiac disease, try to lower intake or gluten by gradually introducing gluten-free foods in your diet. For instance, traditional breads can be replaced with gluten-free breads, or you can buy rice and beans in place of gluten containing grains.

To put all the above into perspective, let's now move on to discussing some delicious gluten free recipes that you can prepare.

# Breakfast Recipes

## Gluten-Free Oatmeal

<u>Serves 2</u>

<u>Ingredients</u>

1 cup whole rolled gluten-free oats

1 teaspoon vanilla extract

1/2 teaspoon kosher salt

1 cup water

1 cup whole milk, almond milk or hemp milk

<u>Directions</u>

1. Over high heat, pour water and milk in a sauce pan then add in vanilla extract and salt. Bring the mixture to a boil.

2. As the liquids boil, pour in gluten-free oats. Stir to mix. After the liquids begin to boil again, lower the heat to simmer the oats while stirring occasionally.

3. Cook for about 15 minutes, or until the oats are creamy and plump and the liquid mixture completely absorbed.

4. At this point, turn off the heat and cover the sauce pan. Allow the oatmeal to cool for around 5 minutes.

5. Then top with maple syrup, blackberries and peaches.

# Ham & Egg Loaded Potato Skins

Serves 4 halves

*Ingredients*

4 medium free-range eggs

A few fresh chives

80g Cheddar cheese

Olive oil

2 rashers of smoked bacon

2 large baking potatoes

*Directions*

1. Preheat the oven to 350 degrees F.

2. Meanwhile, prick the potatoes and pop them on the oven shelve until cooked through. After about 1½ to 2 hours, remove from oven and let cool on a wire rack.

3. Then chop the bacon and add it to a hot pan along with oil. Sauté the bacon until golden and crispy and then tip it into a mixing bowl.

4. Now half the potatoes lengthwise and scoop out the center. Leave about 5 millimeter edge. Add half of the scooped flesh to a bowl.

5. Then finely chop the chives and grate the cheese. Add a third of the cheese and most of the chives to a bowl.

6. Season with black pepper and sea salt then mash the mixture together.

7. Put the potato skins on a baking tray then add a spoonful of filling to each potato. Make a well for the eggs too.

8. Now crack the eggs into the potato and sprinkle with the rest of the cheese. Bake until the egg is cooked and soft, in about 12 minutes.

9. Top with chives and enjoy.

# Hash with Poached Eggs

<u>Serves 4</u>

*Ingredients*

1 ounce Parmesan cheese, shredded

4 large eggs

1 tablespoon white vinegar

2 tablespoons fresh parsley, chopped

2 tablespoons chives, thinly sliced

2 cups seeded tomato, chopped

1/2 teaspoon black pepper, ground

1/2 teaspoon kosher salt

1 cup green beans, trimmed

1 cup yellow squash, diced

1 cup diced zucchini

1 teaspoon dried herbes de Provence

1 cup sliced small red potatoes or fingerling

1 cup sweet onion, chopped

4 teaspoons olive oil

<u>Directions</u>

1. Over medium heat, warm a large non-stick skillet and add in oil, and then swirl to coat.

2. Now add in herbes de Provence, potatoes and onions, and then spread the mixture in a single layer. Cook without stirring for 4 minutes, to have the potatoes lightly turn brown.

3. Then lower the heat to medium and now stir in 3/8 spoon pepper, salt, beans, yellow squash and zucchini.

4. When ready, remove from heat and cover the pan, and then allow it to rest for 5 minutes. Then stir in the parsley, chives and tomato.

5. To a large skillet, add in water up to $2/3^{rd}$ full and bring it to a boil. Then lower the heat to simmer, and then stir in vinegar.

6. Now in a custard cup, break each of the 4 eggs and then pour gently into the pan.

7. Cook for around 3 minutes, and then use a slotted spoon to remove the eggs from the pan.

8. At this point, sub-divide the mixture into 4 plates and top each with an egg.

9. You can use the remaining Parmesan cheese and 1/8 teaspoon pepper to sprinkle on eggs.

# Avocado & Bacon Muffins

<u>Serves 12</u>

*Ingredients*

Salt & pepper

1/2 teaspoon baking soda

1/2 cup coconut flour

1 cup coconut milk

2 cups avocado

4 eggs

6 short cut bacon rashers

1 small onion

*Directions*

1. Preheat the oven to 350 degrees F and then use coconut oil to grease 12 muffin cups.

2. Finely dice the bacon and onion and brown the two ingredients in a fry pan.

3. Meanwhile, use a fork to mix the eggs and avocado together and then stir in milk.

4. Follow with salt, pepper, baking soda and coconut floor and mix well to break up all lumps.

5. Now fold through the 3 quarters of the onion and cooked bacon mixture.

6. Then divide the mixture between the 12 muffin cups and top with the reserved onion and bacon.

7. Bake the cups into the preheated oven for about 20 minutes. Once cooked through, cool and remove the dish from the cups.

8. You can serve immediately or keep chilled in the fridge for outdoor breakfasts.

# Portobello Breakfast Bakes

<u>Serves 2</u>

*Ingredients*

Salt & pepper

2 tablespoons parsley, chopped

4 slices bacon

2-4 large eggs

2 Portobello mushroom caps

1 tablespoon coconut oil or olive oil

*Directions*

1. Preheat your oven to 400 degrees F and then use coconut or olive oil to lightly grease a baking dish.

2. Remove the steps from mushrooms using a knife, to create a small bowl shape.

3. Put the mushroom cups into the baking dish with the right side up and bake for about 5 minutes. Remember to flip upside down and then bake for another 5 minutes.

4. Meanwhile, prepare the bacon. Use an aluminum foil to line a baking sheet and then position the bacon strips in a single layer of the baking sheet. Bake the bacon for 10-15 minutes until done.

5. Once done, remove the caps from heat and then crack 1-2 eggs in each; and return the mushrooms and eggs into the oven.

6. At this point, bake these for additional 10-15 minutes for the egg whites and yolks to be cooked as desired.

7. Then let the bacon to cool down before cutting it into bite sizes. To serve, sprinkle the bacon bits and eggs with parsley.

# Classic Breakfast Casserole

Serves 2

*Ingredients*

Salt, pepper

5 eggs

1/8 teaspoon chili flakes

1 garlic clove, minced

1 teaspoon olive oil

1 oz bacon, cut

250 g ground turkey

½ red onion, chopped

½ yellow pepper, sliced

1/2 red pepper, sliced

1 cup broccoli florets

1 cups cauliflower florets

*Directions*

1. First preheat your oven to around 350 F; and line a baking sheet with baking paper.

2. Then put the broccoli florets, cauliflower, onion and the peppers on the baking sheet; and bake them for 15 minutes to soften.

3. Meanwhile, heat olive oil in a skillet and cook the bacon over medium heat for around 2 minutes or so.

4. Add in ground turkey and brown it too. Then add in chili flakes and garlic. Season and combine fully with the baked veggies.

5. At this point, beat eggs with the ground pepper and salt in a small bowl. Once well blended, set aside.

6. Then add the meat mixture to two oven-safe gratin dishes or to a 4×8-inch casserole dish.

7. Add in the egg mixture and mix well. Bake the final mixture for around 30 minutes until eggs are set.

8. Allow the dish to cool for 5 minutes and then serve.

## Brown Fried Rice Breakfast-Style

*Servings: 2*

*Ingredients*

Salt

4 cups of water

1 cup of short-grain brown rice (or 3 1/2 cups cold cooked brown rice)

1 tablespoon untoasted sesame oil or peanut oil

4 scallions, sliced thinly

1 tablespoon rice wine vinegar

1 tablespoon soy sauce, plus more for serving

2 cups chopped spinach

2 eggs, beaten lightly

Fresh ground pepper

Hot sauce

*Directions*

1. In a medium saucepan, combine the rice with the water and bring to a simmer. Cover and cook the rice over low heat until tender, about 30 minutes; drain.

2. In a large, nonstick skillet, heat the sesame oil until shimmering. Add the scallions and cook over moderate heat until tender, 2 to 3 minutes. Stir in the cooked brown rice, vinegar and soy sauce and cook until rice is heated through, about 3 minutes. Add the spinach and cook until wilted, 2 to 3 minutes longer.

3. Push the cooked rice mixture to the sides of the skillet and add the lightly beaten eggs to the middle, stirring until cooked, 1 minute. Mix the eggs with the rice. Season with salt and pepper and serve hot with soy sauce and hot sauce.

## Almond Vanilla Scones

Serves: 12

*Ingredients*

3 cups (300 g / 10 ½ oz) almond meal

¼ cup (2 fl oz) macadamia nut oil or cold pressed olive oil

1 tablespoon honey or organic maple syrup

2 teaspoons vanilla bean paste

2 free range eggs

vanilla jam to serve

*Directions*

Preheat your oven to 150 C / 300 F.

Combine almond meal and baking powder

Add the oil, honey, vanilla and egg.

Mix into a soft sticky dough

Dust your working surface with a little almond meal

Place over the scone dough and flatten out to 3 cms thick

Cut into small rounds and place onto a baking tray

Bake for 20 – 25 minutes or until golden and your scones are cooked through

Remove from the oven and cool

Serve alone or with your choice of whole fruit jam.

# Lunch Recipes

## Chinese Chicken Salad

<u>Servings: 4</u>

*Ingredients*

2 tablespoon rice vinegar

1 tablespoon peanut oil

1 tablespoon sesame seeds

1 tablespoon hoisin sauce

4 cups mesclun or torn romaine lettuce

2 cups cooked chicken, chopped

3½ ounce Enoki mushrooms

1 can slice water chestnuts, drained

3 scallions, sliced into thin round

1 rib celery, finely chipped

1 teaspoon sesame oil

1 teaspoon mustard powder

12 square wonton wrappers

½ teaspoon sriracha sauce, optional

Directions

1. Preheat your oven to 350 degrees F.

2. Meanwhile, start cutting the wonton wrappers into strips that measure ½ inches. Then position them on a non-stick baking sheet.

3. Coat the strips with cooking spray and then bake them in the preheated oven for 5 minutes; or until lightly browned and crispy.

4. In a large salad bowl, combine celery, scallions, water chestnuts, mushrooms, chicken and lettuce.

5. Then in a separate bowl, whisk together sriracha sauce mustard powder, sesame oil, hoisin sauce, sesame seeds, peanut oil and vinegar.

6. Pour this sauce over the vegetables and chicken and toss to blend. When done, top with the crisp wonton skins. Serve and enjoy.

# Mediterranean Fish

*Ingredients*

Serves 4

Salt and pepper

1 tablespoon lemon juice

1/4 cup olive oil

1/4 cup capers

5 ounce pitted kalamata olives

1 onion, chopped

1 large tomato, chopped

1 tablespoon Greek seasoning

4-6 ounce fillets halibut

Directions

1. First preheat your oven to 350 F degrees.

2. Then put the halibut fillets on an aluminum foil and use Greek seasoning to season.

3. Now mix together pepper, salt, lemon juice, olive oil, capers, olives, onion and tomatoes in a bowl.

4. At this point, spoon the tomato onion mixture over the fish, then seal all the edges using a foil to create a large packet.

5. On a baking sheet, put the packet and bake it in the preheated oven for about 30 to 40 minutes.

6. Once the halibut can flake easily, remove from the oven and serve.

# Tandoori Tofu

Serves: 6

*Ingredients*

6 tablespoons sliced cilantro or scallions

2/3 cup plain yogurt, non-fat

2 14-ounce packages tofu, water-packed and drained

1 tablespoon lime juice

1 tablespoon garlic, minced

3 tablespoons olive oil, extra-virgin

1/4 teaspoon turmeric, ground

1/2 teaspoon coriander, ground

1/2 teaspoon cumin, ground

1 teaspoon salt, divided

2 teaspoons paprika

*Directions*

1. Over medium-high heat, preheat your grill and continue preparing the other ingredients.

2. In a small bowl, mix together paprika, turmeric, coriander, cumin and ½ teaspoon salt.

3. Then in a skillet, heat some oil over medium heat, and add in the spice mixture, lime juice and garlic. Stir well. Cook for about a minute until it's sizzling and fragrant, and then remove from heat.

4. Now cut the tofu block crosswise preferably into 6 slices and pat dry it. Brush both sides of the sliced tofu using 3 tablespoons of spiced oil.

5. Then sprinkle the tofu with a ½ teaspoon of salt. Reserve some of the remaining spiced oil.

6. Now oil the grill rack, and then grill the tofu for about 2-3 minutes, or up until the grill marks are heated trough.

7. In a small bowl, mix the reserved spiced oil with yoghurt. Finally serve the grilled tofu with yoghurt sauce and garnish with cilantro or scallions.

# Mayo Steak Salad

<u>Serves 3</u>

*Ingredients*

1 tablespoon olive oil, organic extra virgin

1/4 cup cilantro

1/2 jicama

1 whole avocado, diced

2 medium tomato (raw), diced

8 oz fresh spinach

1 tablespoon Nanak ghee

8 oz steak

<u>For dressing</u>

Sea salt and pepper

1 tablespoon olive oil

Juice of 3 to 4 limes

*Directions*

1. Season the steak with salt and pepper and then melt ghee over medium-high heat in a cast iron skillet.

2. Then fry the steak for around 4 minutes, flip and cook the other side for 3-4 minutes.

3. Now remove the steak from heat and let it cool down for around 10 minutes. Once cool enough, slice it thinly.

4. Meanwhile, toss the veggies in a large bowl and start to make the dressing. Simply juice the limes in a bowl and whisk in olive oil. Season the ingredients with some pepper and salt.

5. To serve, top the salad with the steak while drizzled with the dressing.

# Sea Vegetable Salad

*Serves: 2*

*Ingredients*

2 drops stevia

¼ cup Apple Cider Vinegar

3 tablespoons raw agave syrup

½ cup dehydrated sour cherries or Inca berries

For Miso dressing:

Few drops of toasted sesame oil

3 tablespoon dark raw agave

¼ cup sesame oil

1 clove garlic

¼ cup chopped ginger

1 lemon juice

¼ cup apple cider vinegar

½ cup Miso shiro

<u>For salad</u>

2 tablespoon black sesame seeds

2 tablespoon white sesame seeds

Bunch watercress, chopped

1 green onion, sliced

1 white radish, julienned

3 beets, julienned

1 tablespoon wakame, soaked and drained

3 tablespoon arame, soaked and drained

*Directions*

1. In a bowl, mix together the apple cider vinegar, raw agave syrup, cherries or berries and sweeten with the stevia.

2. Soak the mixture for about 1 hour, and then drain and set it aside.

3. Now prepare the ingredients for Miso dressing. Just mix them together in a blender and then set aside once ready.

4. To make the salad, mix together all the salad ingredients in a bowl apart from the sesame white and black seeds.

5. Then combine the Miso dressing and sour cherries by hand and stir to combine.

6. Serve garnished with sesame seeds.

# Kale and Fruit Salad-snack

Serves 2-3

Ingredients for the salad:

1/2 a red onion, very thinly sliced

2 bunches kale, or 6 packed cups of baby kale

6 Medjool dates, pitted

1/3 cup whole hazelnuts

For the dressing

5 tablespoons toasted hazelnut oil

Pinch of coarse salt

1 Medjool date

4 tablespoons orange juice, freshly squeezed

2 tablespoons Apple Cider Vinegar

Directions

1. Heat the oven to 375 degrees F. Put hazelnuts into a baking dish and roast for about 7-8 minutes, or until the skin darken and begin to split.

2. Then move the nuts while still hot, steam for 15 minutes while wrapped into a kitchen towel

3. Once cool enough, squeeze and twist around firmly to remove the skin, but while still wrapped into towel.

4. In a food processor, put the hazelnuts and pulse them until fully mixed and finely chopped. Set it aside to top the salad.

5. Wash, dry and chop the kales and then put into a large bowl. Slice the onion thinly and add into the bowl.

6. Prepare the dressing by combining the ingredients for dressing in the blender apart from the oil. Puree the mixture to break down the dates and then drizzle the oil in a steady stream to emulsify the dressing.

7. At this point, toss the kale and onion mixture along with the orange-hazel nut dressing together. Then move to a platter bowl and sprinkle with the hazelnut and dates mixture.

## Quinoa Burgers

*Serves: 1o*

*Ingredients*

1 medium shallot, peeled and roughly chopped

2 cloves garlic, peeled and roughly chopped

1 15-ounce can garbanzo beans, drained and rinsed

1 1/2 teaspoons kosher salt

Juice of 1 medium lemon (about 3 tablespoons)

3 eggs (180 g, out of shell) at room temperature, beaten

1 cup fresh gluten free bread crumbs

3/4 cup (75 g) gluten free old-fashioned rolled oats

2 cups cooked quinoa, cooked in vegetable stock according to package directions (I used red quinoa but it's all the same aside from the obvious (color))

3 to 4 carrots, peeled and shredded (125 g)

3 to 4 tablespoons ghee (or extra virgin olive oil), for frying

*Directions*

1. Preheat your oven to 300°F. Line a rimmed baking sheet with unbleached parchment paper and set it aside.

2. In the bowl of a food processor, place the chopped shallot and garlic and pulse until finely minced. Add the garbanzo beans, the salt and the lemon juice, and pulse until mostly smooth. Add the eggs and pulse to combine. The mixture will have become relatively thin. Add the bread crumbs and rolled oats, and pulse until the mixture begins to come together. Transfer the mixture to a large bowl, add the quinoa and shredded carrots, and mix to combine well. Cover the bowl and place in the refrigerator until the mixture thickens and becomes firmer (about 15 minutes or up to overnight).

3. Remove the bowl from the refrigerator, uncover it, and, divide the mixture into 10 separate burger patties. Moisten hands with cool water as often as necessary to prevent the mixture from sticking to your hands. Place each shaped patty on a paper towel and blot it dry.

4. Heat 2 tablespoons of ghee in a large, heavy-bottom saute pan over medium heat until the ghee is melted

and begins to shimmer. Place as many patties in the pan as will fit without touching one another and fry until golden brown on the underside (about 3 minutes). Flip the patties and fry until golden brown on the other side (another 2 to 3 minutes). Remove the patties to the prepared baking sheet. Repeat with the remaining patties, using the remaining ghee as necessary.

5. Place the baking sheet with the burgers on it in the preheated oven and bake for about 10 minutes, or until mostly firm to the touch. Serve warm.

# Egg Salad Sandwich

*Serves: 4*

*Ingredients*

9 hard-cooked eggs, peeled, whites chopped, 3 yolks crumbled, remaining yolks reserved for another use

1/3 cup mayonnaise, plus more for spreading

1 medium stalk celery, cut into 1/4-inch dice

1 teaspoon Dijon mustard

1/4 teaspoon Madras curry powder (optional)

Coarse salt and freshly ground pepper

8 slices whole-grain bread

1 small head radicchio

1 small bunch arugula, trimmed (optional)

*Directions*

1. Mix whites, yolks, mayonnaise, celery, mustard, and curry if desired.

2. Season with salt and pepper.

3 .Spread mayonnaise on 4 slices bread.

4. Top each with radicchio, egg salad, and arugula if desired. Sandwich with remaining bread.

# Dinner Recipes

## Prosciutto-Wrapped Basil Shrimp

<u>Serves 4</u>

*Ingredients*

10 very thin slices prosciutto

1/8 teaspoon black pepper, freshly ground

1/4 teaspoon red pepper flakes

1/2 teaspoon kosher salt

1/2 teaspoon lemon zest

1 teaspoon extra-virgin olive oil

1 tablespoon fresh basil, chopped

20 large frozen peeled deveined shrimp, thawed

8 lemon wedges, optional

Cooking spray

*Directions*

1. First preheat the broiler.

2. Then mix together black pepper, red pepper flakes, salt, zest, olive oil, basil and shrimp. Combine well and set aside.

3. On a large work surface, lay the prosciutto slices then cut each into half lengthwise.

4. Then wrap the prosciutto pieces around each shrimp, but leave the tail hanging out.

5. Thread the shrimp on an 8-inch skewer and repeat the process for the rest of the shrimp to make 4 skewers with 5 shrimp each.

6. Put the skewers on a broiling pan that is greased with cooking spray. Broil the prosciutto-wrapped shrimp for about 2 minutes on each side.

7. Serve the dish hot with lemon wedges if you like.

# Black-Bean Chili with Winter Squash

<u>Serves 6</u>

*Ingredients*

1/4 teaspoon salt

1 medium winter squash

1/2 teaspoon dried oregano

1 /4 teaspoon chipotle chile powder

1 teaspoon chili powder

1 (4.5-ounce) can mild green chiles, chopped

1 (28-ounce) can diced tomatoes, un-drained

2 cups fat-free, less-sodium vegetable broth

2 (15-ounce) cans black beans, rinsed and drained

3 garlic cloves, minced

1 medium yellow bell pepper, diced

1 large chopped onion

1 tablespoon olive oil

*Directions*

1. Over medium heat, add oil, onion and bell pepper and cook for about 5 minutes, stirring often.

2. Once soft, add in garlic and cook for another minute. Stir in oregano, chipotle powder, chili powder, green chiles, tomatoes, broth and beans.

3. Simmer for 10 minutes while covered. Then uncover and cook for another 10 minutes.

4. Now cut the squash in half, remove the seeds then pierce with a fork a number of times. Place in a heat-proof dish along with ¼ inch water.

5. Using plastic wrap, cover with and microwave on high until tender, or for 8 minutes.

6. Then allow to cool until safe to handle. Use a small sharp knife to peel the squash and cut into ½ inch chunks.

7. Stir the squash chunks into the bean mixture and cook for about 5 minutes. Season with salt and serve warm.

# Indian Mushroom Curry

<u>Serves: 3</u>

*Ingredients*

1 teaspoon Garam Masala

Pinch of turmeric

¾ teaspoon red chili powder

2 -3 tablespoons Oil

½ teaspoon cumin

¼ teaspoon mustard

2 sprigs mint or curry leaves

1 green chili slit

1 teaspoon ginger garlic paste

1 tomato chopped

¾ cup chopped onions

¼ cup green peas or cashews

10 to 12 white button mushrooms

Salt to taste

*Directions*

1. First, slit the green chilies, chop the onions and soak the cashews. Then drain and set aside.

2. In a pan, heat oil along with mustard and cumin and allow to splutter. Then add in mint or curry and green chili and fry the mixture to obtain a sizzling aroma.

3. Add in garlic ginger paste and fry for 1-2 minutes to obtain a good aroma. Then add in the onions, and a sprinkle of salt, and fry until the mixture turns brown. Chop the mushrooms as the onion fry.

4. Then add in tomato puree and sauté until the raw smell goes off and the moisture dries up. If using tomatoes, add chopped ones and fry until they turn mushy and later dry.

5. Now add in garam masala, turmeric, curry leaves and red chili powder; then fry for 1 minute or until the raw smell is gone.

6. Meanwhile, wash the mushrooms under a bowl of water, but don't soak them. Only cut them when

you're to add the curry to prevent discoloring. If desired, get rid of the hairy part, or leave it intact.

7. Drain the cashews off water and add them into the green peas. Fry the mixture on high for about 2 minutes.

8. Add in chopped mushrooms, salt and cashews. Cover the contents and cook on a low flame for around 2-3 minutes to fully cook the mushrooms and let out moisture.

9. Continue to cook until water evaporates then season with a teaspoon of lemon and some salt if you like. Serve with rice and ghee.

# Ground Beef Stroganoff

*Serves 4-6*

*Ingredients*

1/2 teaspoon black pepper

1/2 teaspoon of sea salt

2/3 cup thick coconut cream

1.5 cup beef stock

1 tablespoon arrowroot powder

4 cloves of garlic

1.5 teaspoon rosemary

1.5 teaspoon thyme

2 tablespoon of tomato paste

1 pound of ground beef

8 ounces of white mushrooms, sliced

1 lb Onion, diced

2 tablespoon of coconut oil or olive oil; extra-virgin

2 tablespoon of butter or ghee

*Directions*

1. Melt some ghee or butter in a skillet along with a tablespoon of coconut oil.

2. Then add in onions and mushrooms and sauté until brown around the edges and slightly softened. Now transfer into a plate.

3. Brown the beef in a tablespoon of oil, until it's no longer pink and then return the mushrooms and onions to the pan.

4. Then add in garlic, rosemary, thyme and tomato paste and sauté for around 3 minutes. After a flavor has developed, you can then reduce the heat to medium.

5. To the meat mixture, sprinkle the arrowroot powder and then stir to completely combine.

6. At this point, add in the beef stock and stir to combine. Then simmer to thicken the sauce for about 5 minutes.

7. Once done, cool for a few minutes and then stir in the coconut cream.

8. When ready, serve over sweet potato noodles, cooked cauliflower rice, or roasted spaghetti squash.

## Baja Butternut Squash Soup

Serves: 10

Ingredients

2 tablespoons chopped parsley or fresh chives, snipped

1/2 cup non-fat plain yogurt

1/4 teaspoon pepper, freshly ground

1 teaspoon sea salt

6 cups vegetable broth

1/8 teaspoon cloves, ground

1/4-1/2 teaspoon chipotle chili, ground

1 teaspoon cumin, ground

1 carrot, chopped

1 small onion, diced

2 stalks celery, chopped

1 teaspoon canola oil

1 1/2 pounds winter squash or butternut

*Directions*

1. First preheat your oven to 350 degrees F. Then cut the squash or butternut into half and seed. Put the squash halves into a baking sheet, with the cut side facing down.

2. Bake the squash for about 45-60 minutes, or until its tender. When it's cool to be handled; scoop out the flesh from the squash.

3. Over medium heat, warm some oil in a saucepan and then add in carrot, celery and onion, and stir evenly to coat.

4. Cover the sauce pan and then cook the mixture under medium low heat for about 8-10 minutes, or until soft. Then stir in the cloves, chipotle, cumin and the flesh squash.

5. Now add in broth, and start to simmer when covered for about 20-25 minutes. When done, the vegetables should appear very tender.

6. With a regular or immersion blender, puree the soup until its smooth, and then season using salt and pepper.

7. Garnish with a sprinkle of sparsely or chives and a drizzle of yoghurt.

# Polenta & Feta Vegetable Medley

Serves: 2

*Ingredients*

2 2/3 cups water

4 tablespoons olive oil

1 cup cornmeal (instant)

salt, pepper

1/2 - 3/4 cup shredded Parmesan (optional, omit if vegan)

1 red onion

1 medium eggplant

2 red bell peppers,

2 cloves garlic, minced

chopped cilantro

1 tablespoon tomato paste

1/4 cup feta, crumbled or diced (optional, omit if vegan)

*Directions*

1. Preheat oven to 400 degrees F.

2. Cut the eggplant, bell pepper, and onion into 1-inch cubes. Add vegetables to a large bowl and toss with garlic, olive oil, salt, and pepper. Add vegetables in a single layer to a lightly greased baking sheet. Cook for 45 minutes, until the vegetables are lightly browned, tossing after 20 minutes.

3. Bring water to a boil with salt in a small pot and add polenta slowly while stirring the mixture. Cook for 3 minutes, remove from heat and add the Parmesan.

4. Add half the vegetables to a food processor. Add tomato paste, and pulse a few times until roughly chopped.

5. Serve vegetables over the polenta and sprinkle with feta and cilantro.

# Sweet Potato & Black Bean Chili

Serves: 2

*Ingredients*

2 teaspoons extra-virgin olive oil

1 small onion, finely diced

1 small sweet potato, peeled and diced

2 cloves garlic, minced

1 tablespoon chili powder

2 teaspoons ground cumin

¼ teaspoon ground chipotle chile

⅛ teaspoon salt, or to taste

1⅓ cups water

1 15-ounce can black beans, rinsed

1 cup canned diced tomatoes

2 teaspoons lime juice

2 tablespoons chopped fresh cilantro

*Directions*

1. Heat oil in a large saucepan over medium-high heat.

2. Add onion and potato and cook, stirring often, until the onion is slightly softened, about 4 minutes.

3. Add garlic, chili powder, cumin, chipotle and salt and cook, stirring constantly, until fragrant, about 30 seconds.

4. Add water, bring to a simmer, cover, reduce heat to maintain a gentle simmer and cook until the potato is tender, 10 to 12 minutes.

5. Add beans, tomatoes and lime juice; increase heat to high and return to a simmer, stirring often. Reduce heat to maintain a simmer and cook until slightly reduced, about 4 minutes.

6. Remove from the heat and stir in cilantro.

# Snack Recipes

## The Chewy Gluten Free

<u>Serves 24 cookies</u>

<u>Ingredients</u>

12 ounces semisweet chocolate chips

1 1/2 teaspoons vanilla extract

2 tablespoons whole milk

1 egg yolk

1 whole egg

1 1/4 cups light brown sugar

1/4 cup sugar

1 teaspoon baking soda

1 teaspoon kosher salt

1 teaspoon xanthan gum

2 tablespoons tapioca flour

1/4 cup cornstarch

2 cups brown rice flour

8 ounces unsalted butter

Directions

1. In a heavy bottom saucepan, melt butter over low heat. Then pour the melted butter into a bowl of a stand mixer.

2. Sift together baking soda, salt, xantham gum, tapioca flour, cornstarch and rice flour in a medium bowl. Set aside.

3. To the bowl with butter, add the sugars and cream together using the paddle attachment on medium speed for around 1 minute.

4. Now add in vanilla extract, milk, egg yolk and whole egg and mix to blend. Then gently incorporate the flour mixture to fully combine.

5. Add in chocolate chips and stir to blend. Keep the dough in the fridge for around 1 hour or until firm.

6. Preheat your oven to 375 degrees F. Meanwhile, shape the dough into 2-ounce balls.

7. Put the balls on parchment-lined baking sheets and bake for about 14 minutes. Put 6 cookies per sheet and rotate the pans after every 7 minutes.

8. Then remove from the oven and cool for about 2-3 minutes. Transfer the cookies to a wire rack to fully cool.

9. Store the snack in mason jars or airtight container.

# Fresh Corn Salad

<u>Serves 4 to 6</u>

*Ingredients*

1/2 cup julienned fresh basil leaves

1/2 teaspoon black pepper, freshly ground

1/2 teaspoon kosher salt

3 tablespoons good olive oil

3 tablespoons cider vinegar

1/2 cup small-diced red onion

5 ears of corn, shucked

<u>Directions</u>

1. Cook the corn in a large pot that has boiling salted water until the starchiness is done, in about 3 minutes.

2. Drain and then immerse the corn in ice water until cool. Then cut the kernels off the cob, while cutting close to the cob.

3. Toss the kernels in a bowl along with pepper, salt, olive oil, vinegar and red onions.

4. The toss in fresh basil, taste and adjust the seasoning accordingly. Serve either warm or cold.

# Soft-Boiled Egg

<u>Serves 1</u>

*Ingredients*

Pepper

Salt

1 large organic egg

*Directions*

1. Fill a small deep-sized saucepan with 4 inches water.

2. Bring it to a boil and then reduce the heat to simmer the water.

3. Then lower in the egg and set the timer to 6 minutes.

4. Once ready, remove the egg then make sure to run it under cold tap for 15 seconds.

5. Then place the egg in an egg cup and then slice off the top third.

6. To serve, season with salt and pepper and enjoy.

# Baked Onion Bhajis

Serves: 8

*Ingredients*

1 tablespoon tomato puree

Extra-virgin olive oil, as needed

1/2 teaspoon coriander, ground

1/2 teaspoon cumin

1 pinch salt

5 tablespoons chickpea flour

5 small onions, sliced 5 mm thick

Enough water

For Spices

1/4 teaspoon chili powder

1/4 teaspoon ginger, ground

1/4 teaspoon cumin, ground

1/2 teaspoon coriander, ground

1/2 teaspoon turmeric, ground

*Directions*

1. First preheat our oven to 200 C; and then line a baking tray using baking parchment.
2. In a frying pan, sweat the onions with some oil for around 6-8 minutes, or until translucent.
3. Now sprinkle the chili powder and stir together, and follow with coriander, ginger, cumin and turmeric. Combine fully and remove from heat.
4. In a medium bowl, mix together coriander, salt, cumin and chickpea flour and then and in tomato puree and onions.
5. Add in a sufficient amount of water to achieve required consistency, to obtain a wet and easy to stir mixture.
6. Now drizzle oil on a tray and add 2 tablespoons of the onion mix for each bhaji. Use the back of the spoon to flatten it slightly.

7. In the preheated oven, bake on the middle shelf for around 20-25 minutes, and then drizzle some oil on top of the bhajis.

8. Bake for 25 more minutes to obtain a golden brown dish. Then serve and enjoy.

## Barbecue Zucchini Chips

Serves: 6-8

*Ingredients*

Olive oil

3 zucchini

½ teaspoon black pepper

½ teaspoon mustard

½ teaspoon cumin

1 teaspoon paprika

1 teaspoon garlic powder

1 tablespoon sea salt

1-2 tablespoon coconut sugar, to taste

1 tablespoon chili powder

## Directions

1. Preheat your oven to 300 degrees F.

2. Combine the cayenne, black pepper, mustard, cumin, paprika, garlic, sea salt, coconut sugar and chili powder to prepare a barbecue spice blend in a small bowl.

3. Slice the zucchini to create 1/8 inch slices, and mist the olive oil over the zucchini slices. Then go on to sprinkle the spice blend over the slices of zucchini and bake for 40 minutes.

4. Take out from the oven, flip the slices and mist some olive oil on the other side. Then sprinkle the spice blend over the other side.

5. Bake for around 20 minutes, but take care not to over-bake.

# Spicy Wedged Sweet Potatoes

*Serves: 4*

*Ingredients*

2 tsp ground cumin

2 tsp chilli flakes

2 tsp sumac

2 tbsp thyme leaves, chopped roughly

2 tbsp rosemary leaves, chopped roughly

3 garlic cloves

zest and juice 1lemon

3 tbsp olive oil

1¼kg sweet potatoes , cut into wedges

*Directions*

1. Heat oven to 200C/180C fan/gas 6. Using a pestle and mortar, bash together the spices, herbs, garlic and some seasoning.

2. Spoon into a large bowl and stir in the lemon zest and juice, and the oil. Add the potatoes and toss together. Arrange, skin-side down, on 2 baking trays and bake for 30–40 mins until soft inside and crisp on the outside.

## Conclusion

We have come to the end of the book. Thank you for reading and congratulations for reading until the end.

I hope you have found the book helpful in your quest for delicious gluten free meals!

www.ingramcontent.com/pod-product-compliance
Lightning Source LLC
Chambersburg PA
CBHW071451070526
44578CB00001B/308